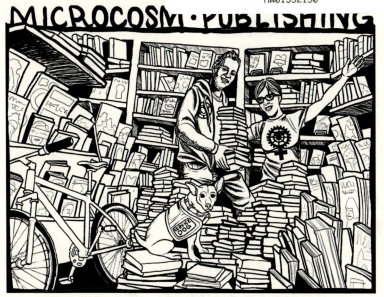

Microcosm Publishing is Portland's most diversified publishing house and distributor with a focus on the colorful, authentic, and empowering. Our books and zines have put your power in your hands since 1996, equipping readers to make positive changes in their lives and in the world around them. Microcosm emphasizes skill-building, showing hidden histories, and fostering creativity through challenging conventional publishing wisdom with books and bookettes about DIY skills, food, bicycling, gender, self-care, and social justice. What was once a distro and record label was started by Joe Biel in his bedroom and has become among the oldest independent publishing houses in Portland, OR. We are a politically moderate, centrist publisher in a world that has inched to the right for the past 80 years.

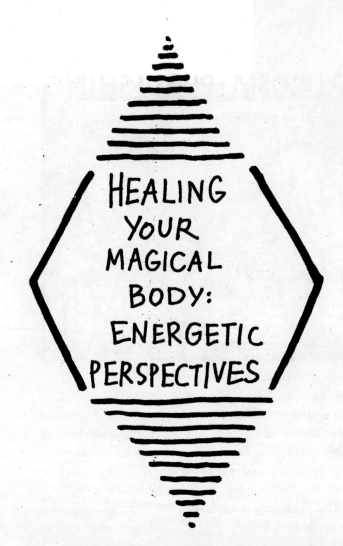

HEALING YOUR MAGICAL BODY: ENERGETIC PERSPECTIVES

© COPYRIGHT 2016 JOJO SHERROW
THIS BOOK WAS MADE WITHOUT COMPUTERS

PIROUETTE PRESS
PO BOX 1001
HUNTINGDON VALLEY
PA 19006

TABLE OF CONTENTS

PREFACE	4
PLANTS TO ENERGETICS	5
INTRODUCTION	6-8
HEALING	9
CREATIVE VISUALIZATION	10
PLANT GUIDES	11-14
S.C.I.E.N.	15-16
EVOLUTION	17-20
DREAM WEAVER LENS	21-22
ENERGY BODY	23-26
BODY COMMUNICATION	27-28
EMPATHING	29
TRIGGERS	30-33
FRAGRANCES	34-36
MEDITATION	37
SLEEP	38-40
DEFINITIONS	41
BIBLIOGRAPHY	42

PREFACE

This is the second book in the Healing Your Magical Body series. The first book has a focus on healing the body with mainly plants, minerals, and food. The newest book titled Energetic Perspectives, is based on research, study, and personal experience with these ideas in the previous four years. Since the year 2012, planet Earth is receiving more photon light from the galactic center of our universe. This in turn is opening up our awareness and bringing in new information for our evolution.

PLANTS TO ENERGETICS

Working with herbs is one step to take when addressing health issues. It's necessary to acknowledge the fact that the problem not only manifests itself as a physical symptom in 3-D reality. All forms of dis-ease exist on the spiritual, mental, and emotional level as well. Some of the ideas proposed in this book will help to connect you more to the planes of existence invisible to most eyes. So you can shift into wholeness.

INTRODUCTION

As human beings, we have the great power to effect a positive change in our bodies and minds that can result in well being. We have the good fortune to be able to respond directly to our own health and our circumstances. We only need certain things like guidance from the plant, animal, and mineral kingdom, both human and non-human allies, teachers, and friends; books, and a positive attitude. There are many ways to approach and address an illness without resorting to allopathic diagnostic procedures or treatments.

The mainstream medical model is not a viable approach for all people. I myself have experienced many medical issues that have <u>only</u> been resolved through alternative methods of healing. Certain types of people will respond very well to alternative therapies. Trust your own intuition to know what is right for you and your body.

If there is any downside to exploring alternatives it is this: you may have to try many different modalities before you find one that works or you may have to combine modalities to resolve a specific health issue.

PLEASE BE PATIENT AND ENJOY THE JOURNEY OF HEALING A PARTICULAR PART OF YOUR BODY AS WELL AS YOUR ENTIRE BEING. AS WE CONTINUE TO QUESTION AUTHORITY, DO OUR OWN RESEARCH, FIND OUT WHAT IS BEST FOR OUR OWN INDIVIDUAL BODIES, MINDS, AND SPIRITS, THE MORE WE CAN CHALLENGE THE HEGEMONY IN PARTS OF OUR SOCIETY. IN THE FUTURE, MORE VARIETY CAN BE OFFERED TO THE NEW GENERATIONS AND THAT WILL BE A REWARD FOR EVERYONE.

IN GOOD HEALTH,
JO-JO SHERROW

HEALING

Sometimes when there is an area of the body that is unwell, part of our awareness is missing from that space. Envision the place of dis-ease and bring a subtle, non-judging awareness back to the body. The awareness feels quiet, calm, and comfortable. It matches the frequency of your essence and your "I AM" presence. This is the energy that facilitates healing in the body and the energetic field around the 3-D body.

Creative Visualization

Creative visualization is to consciously create an image or images in our mind's eye. If we can think of a shiny red apple, this is a form of visualizing. We can improve our skills by creating incrementally more complex imagery. When we do this, our right brain becomes engaged and activated. This part of the brain is instrumental for healing and regenerating the body. We can visualize various shapes, colors, symbols, and sounds to bring our bodies back into alignment.

PLANT GUIDES

THERE ARE MANY OPPORTUNITIES HERE ON PLANET EARTH TO EXPERIENCE THE SAGE WISDOM OF NON-HUMAN GUIDES. THESE GUIDES MAY COME TO US IN THE FORM OF WILD ANIMALS, OUR PETS, ROCKS, LIGHT BEINGS, AND PLANTS.
PLANTS HAVE THEIR OWN SPECIFIC COMMUNICATION THAT OUR RIGHT BRAIN IS ABLE TO TRANSLATE, THEN SEND US THE MESSAGE IN OUR OWN LANGUAGE. BE PATIENT WITH YOUR RELATIONSHIP WITH PLANT COMMUNICATION. CERTAIN PLANTS WILL SPEAK TO YOU

IF YOU GIVE THEM A CHANCE. THEY WON'T SPEAK ALL THE TIME OR SPEAK ON COMMAND. HOWEVER, WHEN THEY DO SAY SOMETHING AND YOU PICK UP ON IT, YOU WILL KNOW IT'S THEM BECAUSE WHAT YOU ARE HEARING DOES NOT SOUND LIKE SOMETHING YOU WOULD SAY TO YOURSELF. THIS TAKES PRACTICE.
A FEW YEARS AGO I HAD A PRETTY BAD CUT* ON MY MIDDLE FINGER, CLOSE TO THE NAIL BED. THE CUT WAS BEING HELD TOGETHER BY ONE OF THOSE BUTTERFLY-TYPE BAND-AIDS SO MORE OF THE SKIN WOULD BE EXPOSED TO THE AIR. AROUND

* THAT WASN'T HEALING

This time I went to a farm in New Hope, PA to pick apples and cherry tomatoes. As I was picking the tomatoes, many were ripe and were getting squished as I picked them. The juice from the tomato got into the cut, burned, and I found myself wincing and getting upset. All of a sudden I hear what sounded like many small voices in my mind," what happened to your finger? Squeeze the tomatoes and put the juice and seeds on your cut." I did. The cut scabbed over the next day. This is one example of how plants can help humans through their wisdom.

TO CLARIFY, ONE NEED NOT GO TO A FARM TO CONNECT TO THE PLANTS. THERE IS AN OPPORTUNITY FOR COMMUNICATION RIGHT IN YOUR KITCHEN WITH THE PRODUCE FROM YOUR SUPER MARKET OR AT THE LOCAL PARK. TREE COMMUNICATION CAN BE ALSO VERY PROFOUND. <u>EXERCISE:</u> PICK ANY TREE THAT IS SOME DISTANCE FROM WHERE YOU LIVE. PRACTICE TUNING INTO THE TREE AS IF YOU WERE CALLING HIM/HER ON THE PHONE. ASK QUESTIONS, RECORD IN A JOURNAL THE ANSWERS, RESPONSES, AND EVEN IMAGERY YOU RECEIVE FROM THIS PARTICULAR TREE. THANK THE TREE.

SCIEN

THE HUMAN RACE AS A SPECIES IS ON AN EVOLUTIONARY FAST TRACK THAT HAS ACCELERATED SINCE 2012. THE GROUP I CALL S.C.I.E.N. IS AND WILL CONTINUE TO PLAY A PIVITOL ROLE IN OUR EVOLUTION. THE ACRONYM STANDS FOR STAR SEEDS, CRYSTAL CHILDREN, INTUITIVE EMPATHS AND NEUROATYPICALS.

THE SCIEN CAN EXPERIENCE LIFE IN THE THREE DIMENSIONAL PLANE OF EXISTENCE IN MYRIAD WAYS THAT ARE DIFFERENT FROM NEUROTYPICAL HUMANS. OUR SENSITIVITIES TO LIGHT, SOUND, COLOR, AND/OR ELECTROMAGNETIC FREQUENCIES ARE A confirmation of our extra sensory perception. We are also more likely to notice thoughts and feelings of others that are unsaid. Like any other group on the planet having a unique experience, the scien serve as a window into the unknown. Certain phenomena that most people don't pay any attention to, (such as the electromagnetic frequencies surrounding our electronic devices) the scien may pick up on or even have a strong reaction as a result of exposure. Their particular view is meant to serve humanity and create positive change for the planet.

WATER, ENERGY, AGRICULTURE

Charles Darwin's research on evolution was appropriate for that particular time in history. For the 21st century, a new approach is necessary. The term "survival of the fittest" is no longer relevant. The evolutionary pioneers in our society are those whose bodies and/or minds are responding directly to the rapidly changing environment post-2012. These people are here to guide the rest of the population on steps to take for humanity to both survive and thrive.

Based on the responses to the changing environment there are three main areas greatly in need of an overhaul. They are water, agriculture, and energy.

1) <u>WATER</u> – Most municipal water, however safe, can contain chlorine or fluoride ions, trace amounts of heavy metals, very minute doses of medications, or pesticides and herbicides. There is a need for a new system of home water filtration. This may include sound, light, or crystals for clearing the water. Access to pure water will improve our health.

2) **AGRICULTURE** - AS WE HEAD TOWARDS THE 22nd CENTURY, IT'S IMPORTANT FOR US TO HAVE EASY ACCESS TO SAFE FOOD. THIS MEANS NON-GMO, ORGANIC, AND ALLERGEN FREE IF NECESSARY. CROPS MUST BE GROWN WITHOUT PESTICIDES OR HERBICIDES AND ANIMALS MUST BE RAISED IN THEIR NATURAL ENVIRONMENT, TREATED WITH DIGNITY AND FED ORGANIC FOOD. IF THIS SYSTEM OF AGRICULTURE IS IMPLEMENTED, THE HUMAN RACE AS WELL AS ALL OF PLANET EARTH WILL RECEIVE GREAT BENEFIT.

3) **ENERGY** - IT IS BOTH UNNECESSARY AND UNSAFE TO USE NON-RENEWABLE RESOURCES AS A SOURCE OF ENERGY. SOLAR, WIND, AND HYDRO POWER ARE EXISTING ALTERNATIVES TO FOSSIL FUEL. NUCLEAR POWER POSES FAR TOO GREAT A RISK AS WE HAVE SEEN IN CHERNOBYL, THREE MILE ISLAND, AND FUKUSHIMA. RATHER THAN BE CONNECTED TO A GRID ELECTRICITY SYSTEM, HOMES OF THE FUTURE WILL BENEFIT FROM SELF-CONTAINED RENEWABLE GENERATORS OF ELECTRICITY. HYDRAULIC FRACTURING (FRACKING) WILL NO LONGER BE AN OPTION,

DREAM WEAVER LENS

WHEN WE FIND OURSELVES WITH A PART OF THE BODY THAT IS WORKING SUBOPTIMALLY, THERE ARE MANY WAYS TO ADDRESS, IMPROVE, HEAL, AND IDEALLY RESULT IN THE ORGAN, TISSUE, OR BODY SYSTEM TO WORK IN A MORE EFFECTIVE AND FUNCTIONAL WAY THAN BEFORE. LET'S LOOK AT THE BODY THROUGH WHAT I CALL THE "DREAM WEAVER" LENS. (INSPIRED BY THE DIGITAL APPLICATION FOR CREATING WEBSITES.) BASICALLY WE HAVE 2 VIEWS, A GRAPHIC VIEW, REFERRED TO AS THE 3-D VIEW AND THE CODE VIEW. THIS CODE VIEW IS THE ENERGETIC, MOSTLY INVISIBLE BACKGROUND INFORMATION THAT INFORMS THE CONTINUAL "3-D PRINTING" OF THE HUMAN BODY.

THE CODE IS THE INPUT. THE INPUT ARE THE EMOTIONS, YOUR RELATIONSHIPS WITH OTHERS, EXPERIENCES, THOUGHTS, AND ENVIRONMENTAL FACTORS. IT ALSO INCLUDES CHEMICALS, DRUGS, MEDICATIONS, AND FOOD. THE COMBINATION OF THESE FORCES/FREQUENCIES HAVE A CERTAIN ENERGY SIGNATURE AND VIBRATION THAT WILL CAUSE THE THREE DIMENSIONAL MANIFESTATION OF SOMETHING. IF WE CAN CHANGE THE CODE WE WILL CHANGE THE 3D REALITY. THE DNA IS ALSO A CODE AND BLUE PRINT FOR THE BODY. DNA CAN BE CODED AND RECODED. ADJUSTMENT OF DNA WITHIN AN ORGANISM IS REAL TIME EVOLUTION.

THE ENERGY BODY

The basis of the light body or energy body is a core pillar or tube of brilliant white light that travels vertically up and down the center of the body. The diameter of the tube can vary from about 1 inch to 2 feet. There are 7 energy centers within the body corresponding to each major gland system.

Each center is associated with a color. From top to bottom they are:

1) PITUITARY – VIOLET
2) PINEAL – INDIGO
3) THYROID – TURQUOISE
4) THYMUS – GREEN
5) SPLEEN – YELLOW

6) ADRENALS - ORANGE
7) GONADS - RED

YOU HAVE ACCESS TO YOUR OWN SEVEN CENTERS, ALSO KNOWN AS CHAKRAS. CHAKRA MEANS WHEEL.

THESE WHEELS ARE SPINNING AROUND THE PILLAR LIKE BEADS ON A SILK STRAND. ALTHOUGH THE WHEELS ARE MOVING FAST, THE CENTERS CONTAIN A BEAUTIFUL STILL POINT. THIS IS A PLACE OF NO POLARITY, NULL MAGNETICS, A VACUUM STATE. THIS IS A CREATIVE SPACE IN THE QUANTUM FIELD OF MULTIPLE DIMENSIONS AND POSSIBILITIES.

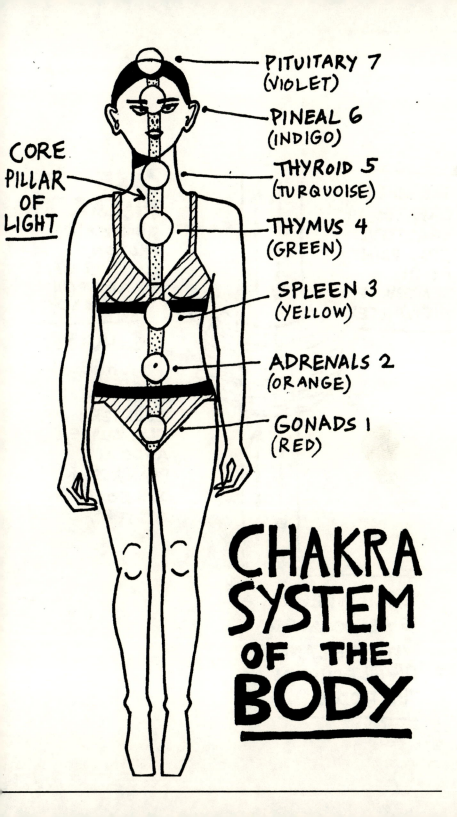

THE WHEEL CREATES A BEAUTIFUL STILL POINT AT THE CENTER OF THE VORTEX.

CORE PILLAR — SHIMMERING PHOTON LIGHT TRAVELS UP AND DOWN VERTICALLY.

CHAKRA (WHEEL): SPINS COUNTER-CLOCKWISE, AS DO ALL PLANETS IN OUR SOLAR SYSTEM.

EACH WHEEL IS ASSOCIATED WITH A GLAND OR GLANDS IN THE BODY.

BODY COMMUNICATION

We as a species are outwardly focused on body language as it relates to our interaction with others. The body's language can also give us clues about our own health issues and areas of the body that need extra T.L.C. EXERCISE: Have a conversation with a part of the body that is hurt or in pain. Touch the body part with your hands and ask what exactly it needs to heal at this moment. Record the answer(s) in a journal. Repeat the exercise daily or weekly for 1 month or a year. Work with a partner and relay the messages you receive to him or her. The answers can be surprising.

SOME SAMPLE QUESTIONS TO ASK YOUR BODY:
1) BASED ON THIS HEALTH ISSUE, HOW IS MY MISSION TO ENCOURAGE, HELP, OR ADD TO THE COLLECTIVE HAPPINESS BEING REVEALED?
2) AM I BEING PRESENTED WITH AN OPPORTUNITY TO TAKE BETTER CARE OF MYSELF AND TO CHECK MY HABITS?
3) IS THERE A RELATIONSHIP IN MY LIFE THAT I MAY HAVE TO EXAMINE MORE CLOSELY?
4) WHEN THE SYMPTOMS FIRST APPEARED, WHAT CHANGES, IF ANY, DID I MAKE IN MY LIFE?

EMPATHING

For certain sensitive individuals, being out in public in the collective field is an opportunity to be empathic. This is when we may pick up on the mental and emotional states of others. It's important to protect ourselves if we are empathing to a degree where we are becoming upset. Recognize what is "their stuff" and what is "your stuff." Silently ask yourself "Is this mine or theirs?" You will receive an answer that resonates with the truth.

TRIGGERS

Q: WHAT DO YOU DO WHEN YOU ARE TRIGGERED?

A: MANY PEOPLE HAVE CERTAIN PEOPLE, SITUATIONS, SOUNDS, + PLACES THAT CAUSE A REACTION WITHIN OUR MINDS AND/OR OUR BODIES. INTUITIVE EMPATHS, INDIGOS, STAR SEEDS, AND THOSE WITH PTSD ARE PARTICULARLY SUSCEPTIBLE TO TRIGGERS. FIRST, HAVE ON HAND (ON THE REFRIGERATOR FOR EXAMPLE) A LIST OF OPTIONS SO YOU KNOW THERE IS A WAY OUT. **STEP 1:** REMOVE YOURSELF FROM THE SITUATION. WALK AWAY FROM THE PERSON, TURN OFF THE TV OR RADIO, SHUT DOWN THE COMPUTER,

A: HANG UP THE PHONE. DON'T PROLONG THE INTERACTION WITH THE TRIGGER.
STEP 2: WHEN YOU ARE SOMEWHERE SAFE (YOUR HOME, ANOTHER ROOM, YOUR CAR, A PUBLIC BATHROOM, ETC.) DO SOME BREATHING EXERCISES. WHEN WE PANIC SOMETIMES THE BREATH IS HELD. 5 SECONDS INHALE, 5 SECONDS HOLD THE BREATH, 5 SECONDS EXHALE. REPEAT 5 TIMES.
STEP 3: RECREATE A HAPPY OR PLEASANT MEMORY IN YOUR MIND. THINK OF ANYTHING THAT WILL RAISE YOUR VIBRATION FROM THAT OF FEAR TO ONE OF JOY.

STEP 4: THINK OF OR PET A CAT OR DOG. PETTING SOFT FUR HAS A CALMING EFFECT ON HUMANS.

STEP 5: HAVE A RELAXATION PLAYLIST PROGRAMMED ON YOUR iPOD. INCLUDE MEDITATIONS, CHANTING, NATURE SOUNDS, AMBIENT MUSIC, OR ANYTHING ELSE THAT WILL RELAX THE NERVOUS SYSTEM

STEP 6: CALL ONE OF YOUR ALLIES. *CAUTION — SOMETIMES WHEN WE FEEL HURT, THERE IS A TENDENCY TOWARDS THE FAMILIAR, EVEN IF IT MAY CAUSE MORE STRESS. REFRAIN FROM CONTACTING CERTAIN FAMILY MEMBERS WHO WON'T BE SUPPORTIVE.

STEP 7: EAT SOMETHING. HAVE HEALTHY, COMFORTING SNACKS LIKE HUMMUS AND CARROTS, MOZZARELLA CHEESE WITH TOMATOES, EDAMAME WITH SEA SALT. IF YOU CRAVE SOMETHING SWEET, TELL YOURSELF THAT YOU WILL LIMIT IT TO A FEW COOKIES, A SMALL SCOOP OF ICE CREAM, OR A FEW SQUARES OF HIGH QUALITY ORGANIC CHOCOLATE. AS YOU EAT THESE FOODS, ALLOW THEIR INTELLIGENCE TO RESET YOUR EMOTIONS AND PLACE YOUR SYSTEM BACK ON THE FREQUENCY OF JOY, HOPE, HAPPINESS, AND CONTENT.

FRAGRANCES

Synthetic fragrances are taxing to the human body and planet earth. These petroleum based compounds are found in:
1) Car trees 2) Air fresheners
3) Scented candles
4) Most cosmetics
5) Perfumes

Since fragrance is a multi-billion dollar industry, these chemicals are ubiquitous.

Replace synthetic fragrance products with:
1) Perfumes, candles, skin care, cosmetics and air fresheners made with essential oils
2) Incense, white sage

SYNTHETIC FRAGRANCES CAN ALSO BE FOUND IN CLEANING PRODUCTS SUCH AS:
1) LAUNDRY DETERGENT
2) DISHWASHING LIQUID
3) CLEANERS
4) SOAPS
5) DETERGENTS

REPLACE WITH:
1) WHITE VINEGAR
2) BAKING SODA
3) LEMON JUICE
4) SUPER WASHING SODA
5) CASTILLE SOAP
6) SMALL AMOUNTS OF LAVENDER OIL AND PEPPERMINT OIL

Q: IF WE ARE EXPOSED TO A SOUP OF CHEMICALS AS WE WALK AROUND IN EVERY DAY LIFE, WHY SHOULD WE BE CONCERNED WITH CHEMICALS ON A PERSONAL LEVEL?

A: OPTING FOR NATURE-BASED, RATHER THAN PLASTIC-CHEMICAL BASED PRODUCTS IS A SMALL STEP THAT OVER TIME WILL LEAD TO A UNIVERSAL CHANGE IN ATTITUDE. AS A PLANET, WE WILL BE MORE AWARE OF THE FACT THAT CERTAIN CHEMICALS CAN BE ENDOCRINE DISRUPTORS. AS EXPLAINED ON PAGE 23 THE ENDOCRINE SYSTEM IS A GATEWAY TO THE CHAKRAS AND ARE VITAL TO OUR HEALTH.

MEDITATION

When we meditate, we can access the theta brain wave state. In this state of 6-7 Hz, we can send effective messages of wellness to various parts of the body. We can direct our DNA to repair any damage that has occured in the code. Our thoughts are subliminal messages. For most of us, quieting the internal dialog is most challenging. Thoughts can be interference or they can be healing. In this state we can receive messages from higher dimensions and from our higher self.

SLEEP

If we are having trouble sleeping at night, there are many different techniques to try for addressing this problem.

1) Make sure your bedroom is completely dark at night. This is a requirement of the pineal gland to make melatonin, the hormone responsible for keeping circadian rhythms.
2) Take herbs: chamomile, valerian, skullcap, passionflower, linden
3) Avoid blue lights (phone, computer, TV) 3 hours before bedtime.
4) Apply lavender oil to your pulse points - wrists, neck, groin, ankles.

5) BE SURE TO GO OUTSIDE AND EXPOSE SOME OF YOUR SKIN TO DIRECT SUNLIGHT FOR AT LEAST 5 MINUTES PER DAY. THIS WILL ALSO HELP RESET YOUR INTERNAL CLOCK.

6) DURING THE DAY, WORK IN NATURAL LIGHT CONDITIONS. LET THE SUN SHINE IN THROUGH THE WINDOWS. AVOID FLUORESCENT LIGHTS IF YOU CAN. CFC (COMPACT FLUORESCENT) BULBS ARE HARSH ON THE EYES AND CONTAIN MERCURY.

7) TAKE DEEP BREATHS THROUGHOUT THE DAY TO CLEAR YOUR LUNGS SO THEY CAN RELAX DURING SLEEP TIME.

8) MUSIC AND SOUND. PLAY A MEDITATION CD, GREGORIAN CHANTS, HINDU KIRTANS, BINAURAL BEATS, OCEAN SOUNDS, BIRD SOUNDS, RAIN + GENTLE STORM SOUNDS, WILDLIFE, CLASSICAL MUSIC, LIGHT DRUMMING, MUSIC BASED ON THE WHOLE TONE SCALE, PENTATONIC SCALE CHROMATIC MUSIC, OR RAGAS. CERTAIN WORLD MUSIC MAY HAVE A CALMING EFFECT ON THE PSYCHE. LISTEN TO MANY DIFFERENT STYLES TO SEE WHICH ONES SUIT YOU - BRAZILIAN, ETHIOPIAN, JAPANESE, KOREAN, RUSSIAN, NATIVE AMERICAN, AFRICAN. THERE ARE MANY POSSIBILITIES.

DEFINITIONS

STAR SEEDS - PEOPLE LIVING ON EARTH WHOSE SOUL ORIGINS ARE ELSEWHERE. THIS DEFINITION MAY CHANGE OVER TIME AS WE RECEIVE MORE INFORMATION ABOUT THIS INTERESTING PHENOMENON.

CRYSTAL CHILDREN - THESE CHILDREN WERE BORN AFTER 2005 AND MAY HAVE A HEIGHTENED LEVEL OF AWARENESS AND CERTAIN SENSITIVITIES.

INTUITIVE EMPATHS - THESE PEOPLE ARE HIGHLY SENSITIVE TO STIMULI AND THE EMOTIONS OF OTHERS.

NEURO-ATYPICALS - THESE PEOPLE DISPLAY A DIFFERENT NERVOUS SYSTEM FUNCTIONALITY THAN THE AVERAGE PERSON. THEY MAY INCLUDE BUT ARE NOT LIMITED TO THOSE WHO HAVE ASPERGERS SYNDROME, THOSE ON THE AUTISTIC SPECTRUM, PEOPLE WITH ADD OR ADHD, AND OTHERS WHO HAVE SO-CALLED "MENTAL ILLNESS."

FURTHER READING

Barbara Lamb
Gwilda Wiyaka
Liza Callen
Julie Loar
Suzanna Kennedy
Louise Hauck
Veronica Entwistle
Meg Benedicte
Nick Redfern
Judy Beebe
Craig Campobasso
Scott Onstott
Meg Blackburn
James Gilliland
Margaret Starbird
Maureen St. Germain
Sarah Starfire
Kae Thompson-Liu
Debi Tripp

SUBSCRIBE!

For as little as $13/month, you can support a small, independent publisher and get every book that we publish—delivered to your doorstep!

www.Microcosm.Pub/BFF

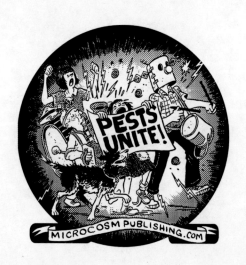